THE VALUE OF COAL: *A WOMAN PERSPECTIVE*

Dr. Brittney Clinton

This book is dedicated to all the women who have endured the pressures of life that transformed you into the diamond you are today.

Don't Quit

When things go wrong, as they sometimes will,

When the road you're trudging seems all uphill,
When the funds are low and the debts are high,
And you want to smile, but you have to sigh,
When care is pressing you down a bit-
Rest if you must, but don't you quit.
Life is queer with its twists and turns,

As every one of us sometimes learns,
And many a fellow turns about
When he might have won had he stuck it out.
Don't give up though the pace seems slow -
You may succeed with another blow.
Often the goal is nearer than

It seems to a faint and faltering man;
Often the struggler has given up
Whe he might have captured the victor's cup;
And he learned too late when the night came down,
How close he was to the golden crown.
Success is failure turned inside out -

The silver tint in the clouds of doubt,
And you never can tell how close you are,
It might be near when it seems afar;
So stick to the fight when you're hardest hit -
It's when things seem worst that you must not quit.

Table of Contents

Introduction

Episode I- "Even Diamonds Start as Coal"

Episode II- "It's Hard to be a Diamond in a Rhinestone World"

Episode III- "Diamonds are only Lumps of Coal that stuck at it no matter how much heat or pressure they faced"

Episode IV- "Perhaps I should just bury myself and become a diamond after thousands of years of intense pressure"

Episode V- "Pressure does two things- burst pipes and creates diamonds. Which one are you?"

Episode VI- "Choose to Shine"

Episode VII- "I eat diamonds for breakfast"

Episode VIII- "Under pressure she became a diamond, under pressure she became unbreakable"

Episode IX- "Don't lose a diamond while chasing glitter"

Episode X- "Don't let someone dim you're light simply because it's shining in their eyes"

Episode XI- "The wasted years, the wasted youth, the pretty lie's, the ugly truth"

Episode XII- "Don't be a hard rock when you really are a gem"

Episode XIII- "Into every woman's life a little diamond should fall"

Episode XIV- "Everybody wants to be a diamond, but very few are willing to get cut"

Episode XV- "A diamond is a chunk of coal that did well under pressure"

Episode XVI- "Some people lose diamonds in search of stones"

Episode XVII- "Start living your life fearlessly; like a diamond"

Episode XVIII- "You can't rush something you want to last forever"

Episode XIX- "Better a diamond with a flaw than a pebble without"

Episode XX- "I love diamond facials; they leave me glowing and refreshed"

Episode XXI- "Be careful who you cast your diamonds too"

Episode XXII- "We are diamonds were gonna shine forever"

Introduction

Women of excellence often go through a diamond in the rough experience which include but not limited to having exceptional character, having potential but lacking polish and refinement, good qualities despite a rough exterior, or one who has good qualities that are often hidden. These seasons of life are meaningful and purposeful prior to going through the rigorous process to become the woman she desires to be. A woman of distinction often looks for ways to condition herself by having daily reflections on what has taken place and what need to be done in order to reach the next major milestone; therefore, she will be able to sit and chat with other woman of valor about what it truly mean to be a diamond in the rough. Success is defined by one's own vision and purpose. My success is not your success. You locate your passion; despite hardships, identify your support circle even if it's one or two, locate individuals who have accomplished and are successful at that same gift that reside within you and just do it. It is not easy, and things will come up that will make you feel like your purpose and vision is dead weight. Think about how a diamond is really formed. The progression to its identity, shape, and form begin seventy-five to one hundred and twenty miles below the earth's surface helps us to understand that this process is deep. Are you willing to fall through the crevice's, run through unseen pipes, burst into existence, and wait for someone to locate your existence and announce the great works you have developed and encountered over time? A diamond endures the pressure and you can too if you really want it! It is in good hope that you find the following personal life experience reflected upon a woman who started life out in a coal mine and chose to reveal the diamonds that were within.

Episode I

"Even Diamonds Start as Coal"

Living in a coal mine mentally was a major challenge. This experience began originally after taking my body under the pressure at a young age carrying and birthing two children. Postpartum after my six week check-up is what they diagnosed me with or any woman that shows emotional distress. I went through the proper protocol in order to get back to where I needed to be. My second round of diagnosis occurred a year later after the birth of my baby boy but this time; it was severe and was suggested that I maintain my mental using prescribed medications in order to return back to school after my six week healing period. I was so hungry to beat the odds and finish my undergraduate degree on time having two children two children a year and two weeks apart. I did as I was told; thought nothing of it and kept it moving. On the bright side; I finished my undergraduate degree on time with two bundles of joy and a husband at that time. It looked as if I completed the perfect life circle by being married, maintaining academic excellence, and being a new mommy of two; however, I remained in a mental coal mine after it all. After finishing college fall 2009, I didn't think no more about the anti-depressant the doctors prescribed me to manage myself; therefore, I kept moving forward. Till this day; I still don't recall the day I stop taking the anti-depressants but I registered to begin my master's degree immediately after. At this point; I was rolling. I was managing it all as a newly wife, mother of two young youngsters, and a graduate student running a certified home daycare. I was at home with children all day, completed the required paperwork for my in home daycare, transported kids to and from the home daycare, and picked up my own children towards the end of the day at a private sitter. I still filled my duties to love and nurture my boys before I went into my zone to work on my coursework for graduate school. I had to experience the sacrifice of detachment from my babies while I completed my coursework nightly between the hours of nine pm to twelve midnight. I though being a married woman; I would have the support of an understanding mate while going through the process but times were challenging and questions like "why would you close the door in they face like that" would arise and I at this point had a selfish mindset and would respond "I have to get my work done, you can handle them for at least an hour".

A woman like myself during my early twenties; still getting to know myself and experience life with all these responsibilities yearn for success and was determined to get it regardless of any circumstances. There were countless nights burning the midnight oil in order to remain on task as a distinguished graduate student. My mind was constantly busy and active; I had no time to think negatively or feel burned out. My body was use to grinding and not sweating at all. At the time; to me, everything had fallen into place being a young African American entrepreneur, working on a master's degree, being an outstanding mother to my boys and a wife at the time. My success was making its own noise and I was climbing the mountain. It had come to my attention after several discussions about the changes that were taking place in the house hold that was causing me to mentally return back to the mental coal mine. I didn't understand it. I thought once I got married; everything and all the previous concerns would go away but somehow they resurface in random moments and confirmations that caused me to seek some spiritual insight on what was taking place. What did I do? I became very observant to every move that was being made but that did not stop my desire to master my coursework for graduate school. The pressure at this point was uncomfortable but bearable. Many times I felt like I had no time to myself because I was running a business, being a mommy, graduate student, and a wife. It got to the point where I would just grab the car keys a leave out the garage door just to ride and get some air. I was accused of doing other things while I was out when I only drove through the city chatting with a close college girlfriend that new the ends and outs of my personal feelings and life challenges. I didn't trust anyone else but her. The mental coal mine became a dark place; a place I never thought I would experience because we count on the happy place in life to last forever. Well it didn't. My diamond in the rough experience began in the blink of an eye; twenty-four hours later, I stood with nothing! I literally was a hard piece of coal.

Episode II

"It's Hard to be a Diamond in a Rhinestone World"

Rhinestones look good too so I'm not throwing shade at all. However, a diamond mindset of a poise woman produces the best quality results; therefore; I will always strive to be the best I could be. Generational curses with the women in my family; I was learning early not to accept anything in a marriage that's not right. Society says that my generation (80's baby) expects a microwave lifestyle like everything suppose evolve quick fast and in a hurry. I discovered that my purpose was to get on track with the help of the village that helped me with my children and keep pressing on. The rhinestone experience was attractive, promising, and overrated! Ladies; I thought I had something going. You could not tell me anything! As I laughed out loud; I began to get back on my feet networking within the community; beginning my journey as a local author in the city of Winston-Salem, NC, and being selected to operate in various leadership roles. Sounds good; huh? It was all good! I felt like a diamond to those who supported me continuously with their powerful words of inspiration and validation to move forward with my future endeavors. That one attractive, promising, and overrated rhinestone that had my heart leaping was becoming a major distraction that began affecting my mental stability. I was beginning to question myself as to why I put so much effort in supporting others in their endeavors when negative backlash was given to me when I was an active platform for the community with my positive and motivated efforts. Going through a rhinestone experience when you deserve a diamond voyage will eventually come to reality when too many disappointments become consistent, unbelievable, and unbearable. Feeling like I was not good enough was the worst feeling when I knew the entire time I was a diamond literally living in a rhinestone world that was fabricated to no end. Once I completed my doctoral studies; I was tired and was ready to enjoy life and become more settled with my two children. The rhinestone world was becoming old to me. I cared less how attractive, promising, and overrated it was; I wanted out.

The rhinestone world was becoming my downfall, a hindrance to what I was really seeking for, and a six year complacent comfort zone that was applying pressure to my mental breakdown. Yes I said it; mental breakdown! My mental was on information overload and did not know how to control it one day out the blue. I encountered uncontrollable crying, panic attacks, and severe depression. While visiting the emergency room several times within a two week time frame; it was mandated that I attend a ten day group therapy session. Listen; I was petrified that someone would see me entering the building were most people say the "crazy" people went for help after having a major episode. I got the courage and made it every day on time with the thought and hope that someone in the building will be helping me. It was hard to get up to get dressed, eat, and do minute activities that required me to associate with other people. My phone would ring and I would just look at it and not answer. I knew that something had happen and I did not know how or why. The ten days spent in group therapy was worth it and I am so glad I sought out professional help.

Each day in therapy; I saw a difference in myself. I recall asking my psychiatrist *"will my appetite ever come back"*? Every question I had was answered with the following reply: *"yes; in due time"*. I learned the importance of my personal bill of rights during this experience as well as how to say the word "no". This process forced me to restructure my priorities and the people I was associating with. If you or anything else was causing me to stress; my mind, body, and soul placed a wall of steal for me to slowly turn around and walk away in the opposite direction. By day 4; I was waking up looking forward to sharing what my goal would be for the day and the things I planned to do that would help me reach my goal. Day four was good day also because I ate the lunch that was provided by the doctor's office and was beginning to feel my strength. The end of the first week included making a family with a select few of my group members that kept one another encouraged and on time for med checks. We all saw one another grow and become better mentally, physically, and socially. A scholar once said; things get worse before they get better and that's exactly how I would compare the Rhinestone experience. With the help of prayer warriors that prayed night and day on my behalf, my support group in group theory, and God alone; I finished knowing that I was a true reflection of a real diamond.

Episode III

"Diamonds are only Lumps of Coal that stuck at it no matter how much heat or pressure they faced"

The lumps of coal that stuck began when I conceived not one child but two children out of wedlock. The pressure of outsiders asking me when my children father and I would get married and how blessed I would be if I just did it for the kids got on my last nerve. No one had a clue that getting married when I became a first time mother was nowhere on my mind because I was still working on my undergraduate degree at Winston Salem State University. I knew at this point that it was possible I would be raising a child alone with the help of family and friends. I was honestly ok with that because my focus was not on what others believed was a failure but focused on the future. I walked the college campus on time for class each day. My classmates knew I was coming to class with my classic bacon cheeseburger, fries, and Pepsi. The heat and the pressure I endured took a toll on me mentally and physically. Entering the campus one morning to check my email in a computer lab where I would meet up with some colleagues and I just wasn't feeling right. I was about four months pregnant with my oldest son. Waffles and orange juice was my breakfast. I felt the need to go to the bathroom and soon as I made a quick right out the lab door towards the bathroom; boom; hit the floor; I passed out. One of my colleagues came to see after me and asked if I wanted the ambulance. The ambulance escorted me off campus and took me to the hospital to check on baby. I was told that my pressure had dropped and to be careful after following up with my primary doctor. The doctor wrote me out for a couple of days but I made sure I was able to submit my assignments and prepare for any upcoming research and assessments.

    I dealt with various lumps of coal that transformed me into the person I am today. I had no time to sit and have a pity party when things failed; I literally got back up and tried again. The heat continues to rise and the pressure was tense. I was that one diamond that stuck together; when broken and crumbled up no matter how much heat or pressure I faced.

Episode IV

"Perhaps I should just bury myself and become a diamond after thousands of years of intense pressure"

Life brought me experiences that the typical young person would have given up on due to the time and dedication that was needed to be successful. I spend ten penetrating years in school while becoming a new mom, wife, and business owner. It was a challenging experience to face the world after being divorced. Even when those around me doubted me; I still saw me reaching my goal to complete graduate school. I was looked and viewed as a rebellious wife. I never understood how people could be so cruel when they never had a clue what was taking place in my life. Every story wasn't meant to be shared when I was married. It has never been good in the African American community to share your thoughts and concerns with relatives while married because it would negatively affect your relationship with your spouse. So no; I never shared anything that took place that made me make the decisions I made. I felt used and abuse because I was younger and had a lot going for myself and was looking for love in all the wrong places. You may ask; why did you marry after you said you were not thinking of marriage? Well; the intense pressure from those individuals that meant the world to me is what caused me to have a change of heart. I also thought that it would change the key factors that hindered me wanting to pursue marriage in the first place. I had no clue that the past experience at a young age would provide so much knowledge and confidence within me today. I buried myself to be a submissive woman and it was darn if you do and darn if you don't.

With all the obstacles; I saw nothing but continued success. I constantly held my head high despite what others had to say; moved in silence and did what I needed to do to reach personal and professional goals. My pressure points were pushed at times where I thought I was going to lose it all; however, I had a community support system that pushed me to run the course and focus on the light that was at the end of the tunnel. One of my sister scholars always reminded me how my work was speaking for me and to trust the fire burning process and in due time; my light will forever shine!

Episode V

"Pressure does two things- burst pipes and creates diamonds.

Which one are you?"

Pressure was becoming a force that was pushing me into my destiny. Every time my back was against the wall in relationships with men or with so-called girlfriends; a lesson was being taught for the next experience that would follow that carried similar characteristics. I caught myself holding everyone down regardless how they treated me and yes I felt like bursting pipes of uncontrollable emotions balled up and released when I just couldn't take it anymore. It took me the longest time to understand that every intention is not meant for good. I recall accepting an opportunity that I thought was heaven sent during a difficult time in life being a single mom trying to make it as a part-time professor and graduate student. I jumped on the opportunity honestly believing that the offer was genuine for my professional development not knowing I would be hood-winked. I faced pressure time after time being a young scholar and recruited to fulfill roles only to look good on paper for others to promote themselves. I had been in the habit of learning to be an effective leader by modeling servant leadership and helping other scholars that express great interest in my ability to be effective within their organization. In my field of expertise (education leadership and management) others immediately assume I knew what to do and how to do while working on coursework and even after the completion of my studies; therefore being left out when I should have been included set a trap to be viewed as not competent to fulfill my roles and responsibilities. The cycle from one opportunity to another was repeating itself and I begin to reflect on what to do next.

Building enough courage to accept the reality of all encounters and know how to engage with other professionals who may or may have not accomplished their goals and interact as if my mind is a blank slate. I know nothing; teach me everything while in reality; I'm well aware and knowledgeable but choose not to share insight because my work speaks for me and continuously illuminates opportunities for others.

Episode VI

"Choose to Shine"

It is up to you to allow your light to shine. I was never the girl that followed the crowd to be involved with anything and everything. I created the path I took because that's what I wanted to do. I was not trying to impress no one but myself. I had already fulfilled the family curse by conceiving not one child but two children. At this point; I had no choice but to beat the odds and shine like a diamond. Doing what others believed to be impossible was my goal because I did not want my children to go through not having their mother inattentive with parent teacher conferences, making ball games and performances, and most importantly, making sure they have the things they need through financial support. I started off continuing my education despite what others thought of me at a young age. I often got *"you so boring, you not living life, you are wasting your younger years, and honey; I don't see how you do it"!* Those words quickly turned into celebratory statements of encouragement being successful (*in their eyes*) at the age of twenty-eight. Everything other thirty-year-old persons are just placing on their to-do list; not to toot my own horn, but I did it along with kids and a major diagnosis of anxiety and depression. It all sounded good until I just told you that I am a mental patient that just earned her doctoral degree at age twenty-eight. What does that tell you? Not the cliché statement *"don't judge a book by its cover"* but success cause some major coal piles that stick closely together to produce a diamond in the rough (*literally*). The best thing that came out of me being medically diagnosed is the mandatory ten-day group therapy session that taught this ole scholar her personal bill of rights and how to effectively learn how to say no. I honestly didn't think it could possibly happen, but I ultimately learned that the mind was a terrible thing to waste. No, I did have a nervous breakdown; my mind was just on information overload and my body was not use to sitting still and just resting.

Some days I felt like associating myself but most days I did not. During this rough stage in my life at age twenty-eight and as accomplished others highlighted I was; I still felt unaccomplished. By the end I finished my ten-day therapy sessions; I humbly accepted that I am indeed successful, understood successful people have pitfalls, and knowing not all pitfalls are noticeable. As I have had the opportunity to share the re-birthing experience; I wake up daily eating diamonds (*success*).

Episode VII

"I eat diamonds for breakfast"

Every morning I wake; I feed my mind quotes that will contribute to my own personal growth. I found quotes that are for inspiration, motivation, leadership, and success. I would place these famous quotes in a generator to launch out on my personal social media sites. Viewers may ask if that's how I feel or is something wrong and little do they know; those are reflections of a successful person. Every feeling or thought does not post as an award winning image. Some images will not truly express what it took for that person to stand and be called Doctor so and so or attorney so and so. Once an individual reach their peak; he or she must continue to feed oneself success. You may retrieve your nutrients through mentoring; sharing your personal experiences, reading motivational text, or embracing your spiritual connection of whom you may worship that keeps you embedded in moving forward. I often tell myself that I have been through the valley before and the man above brought me out and I know he will bring me out again in his timing. I sat for days wanting to begin writing a book reflecting my past experiences and how I was able to obtain and maintain success with life's obstacles. I knew one day I would get the courage to share my experiences to help the next woman seeking for knowledge about how success is obtained and maintained. Eat diamonds for breakfast ladies and gentlemen! Every morning; you should be place a nice sweet diamond ice cube in your coffee and get the day started! Note that it will not be easy but each day; your goals and aspirations will come to life with consistency and determination. What will you eat for breakfast queens?...Diamonds!

Episode VIII

"Under pressure she became a diamond, under pressure she became unbreakable"

There was many times where I wanted to break because I could not win for loosing. Year after year eating diamonds for breakfast, lunch, and dinner became overwhelming. I had support all around me pushing me to bring my vision to life. I had to make some decisions that were hard to make in order for me to keep my sanity. I found myself so caught up in the situation; I was losing the value of myself. I honestly thought everyone I built a friendship and relationship with valued the true meaning of friendship and time after time their actions taught me otherwise. I recall building professional relationships with others by providing my insight and expertise on various tasks and ideas to later find out that the opposite party intentions were all to benefit them. In professional settings you are required to some extend to build collaborative relationships in order to be identifying as a team and a team player. When I tell you that I have a brick wall that strongly avoid anything that's contaminated. At this point in life; I do not allow others emotions, attitudes, values, perceptions affect my day, time, or daily routine. I accept others for who they are and where they are. I do not frown upon their perceptions of life and reality.

With life lessons that came from different angles; personally, and professionally, I have learned to endure the pressure that is bestowed upon me in any circumstances through prayer, meditation, and faith. Overcoming depression and anxiety can be a struggle if you do not have the proper ingredients to maintain a growth mindset. It's easy to fall into depression when things upset you or not going the way you planned but make the choice to do things that will not get you to the point where you allow it to control you or your destiny.

Episode IX

"Don't lose a diamond while chasing glitter"

We as individuals often chase everything that looks good. Ladies; we chase men, friends, opportunities, and the latest trends thinking we have something. We jump through hoops and bounds to stay on top to later find out that what we worked so hard for was full of gold glitter. Gold glitter looks nice and stand out and have you feeling like you hit the jack pot but overtime you begin recognizing the diamond that you are and you just settling for comfort. I been there and done that. Just because it seems as if I've attained many achievements does not mean I have not made mistakes that have caused me to reflect on the times where I was chasing opportunities to be disappointed and look upon as a woman that has lost her substance. Well, guess what?..I did on more than one occasion. I have come to accept that educated, talented, and individuals of valor serve others on major platforms and have major issues and doctor diagnosis.

    I chose to break the status quo as an African American successful woman and seek professional help when I was unable to help myself. I knew I had too much to lose; especially the value of my education and the aspirations I had declared to achieve by impacting the lives of others; I had to get seek professional help. I want other women to accept and understand that every moment will not be the perfect moment. I was busy chasing and not caring for my own health; which is why I ended up taking a mandatory ten-day sabbatical ordered by my physiatrist. To be honest; those where the best ten days that changed my life and my newly growth mindset. I met other distinguished career driven women and men of all nationalities; which help me cope even better seeing it in reality that there are others out in the world that's struggling with life after a major pitfall. I share that with you so that you feel comfortable asking for help if you are ever placed in a position where you know within yourself that you can't do it alone and need professional help. I no longer immediately chase things that look like gold. I search for the proper resources to make it worth earning a diamond experience in the end.

Episode X

"Don't let someone dim your light simply because its shining in their eyes"

Do not belittle your gifts because you don't have the support you thought from your so-called friends, constituents, and professional colleagues. Your initial experience may be something simple as being honored at a banquet that has a table reserved just for you and your supporters. Everyone asks you to save them a ticket. You announce the price of the tickets and you end up paying for most of the tickets to give to those who really wanted to come but did not have the funds at that moment to purchase a ticket. Your table was full and you were thankful for those who attended but your ride or die professional colleague was not there and did not make it to the previous event either due to an emergency the day of. You begin thinking about if you did something to the person, was it really something that came up, or if they are really in your corner. Please don't be blind to the fact that once you have decided to pursue a growth mindset and things begin to fall into place; everyone will not be onboard. It's ok. Don't stop shinning and implementing your talents because others are not supporting you or telling you *"you doing too much"*. You keep writing your goals and checking them off the list as you go along. At some point; you will be connected with the right people at the right time that will help you pursue your vision and contribute to your success voluntarily. Sometimes you have to promote yourself with what you have and gain appropriate resources during the process that will land you to implement what you have to offer on a larger scale.

Know that you are worthy to be recognized for the hard work you have put in overtime impacting the lives of others. With or without supporters; understand that your expertise in the areas you are gifted are needed to help someone else; therefore, do your thing and don't worry about who's distracted by your light. Most importantly; make sure you are setting the example by supporting others during your journey.

Episode XI

"The wasted years, the wasted youth, the pretty lies, the ugly truth"

Years and years had gone by before I fully accepted that I was not satisfied with a few family relationships. I wanted questions answered, heart to heart moments, and clarity as to why things transpired the way they did up into adulthood. During the course of my ten day group therapy sessions; I had to write down the relationship I had with my mother, father, and siblings in detail. I had to retell stories about how we engaged with one another from then to now. It was a hard pill to swallow because as I was describing the relationship I had with each; I recognized how emotionally drained I was. I was truthful as to how I use to treat my brothers so selfishly when it came to me sharing things with them. I recall others asking when I was a child, *"why do you treat your brothers like that?"* Back then I did not know I was setting myself up to be emotionally disturbed as an adult and the relationship I have with my siblings. I did not know I was going to grow up being so passionate about the growth of others personally and professionally. I immediately broke down and felt guilty for mistreating them when we were younger. I prayed that they would forgive me and embrace my outreaches during our adulthood.

Happy connecting! Connecting with my siblings after therapy was a heart to heart. I shared with them the truth about how I recognize the wasted years, wasted youth, the pretty lies, and avoided the ugly truth. I humbly apologize for my behavior and asked for their forgiveness. They responded and told me it was ok and I didn't know what I was doing at the time due to me being raised along in grandma's house. My brothers think about me every holiday and special occasion and I will always be grateful and cherish the moments. They did not have to choose to build a relationship with me after being so disconnected over the years because I thought it was all about me but they did and I'm grateful.

Episode XII

"Don't be a hard rock when you really are a gem"

Life will bring moments where you second guess your own potential due to not executing at your best at one task. You will have days where you don't feel like a professional career driven entrepreneur and that's ok.

Don't be so hard on yourself when you are made to shine always like a gem. When you are behind closed doors in sweat pants, a messy bun, and a cup of Starbucks mapping out your next move; you still a gem baby! Take time to take care of yourself and your mental. You don't have to look like America's top model whenever your own the grind. Granted; it's encouraged to look respectable always because you never know who you may encounter on that day. While being involved with various platforms within the community; I am constantly running into individuals I've met in professional settings; therefore, I make sure I'm in place from head to toe. I'm not beat to the Gods but a little lip gloss, some earrings, jeans and a shirt will get the job done. Just because I am *"Dr. Clinton or Dr. C"* does not mean I have to dress in black, white, navy, and grey professional attire always. I recall running into one of my sister scholars in New York and Company in the mall and she was chilling in her sweat pants and t-shirt with no make-up. I have always payed close attention to the way she dressed, the way she carried herself while handling her personal life (very quiet and personal), and most importantly, her approach to the education profession. While observing and researching her path to success over time; it taught me so much about being hard on myself when things are not taking place when I needed it too the most. My community of support often remind me despite of life tragic events that I am *"Dr Clinton"* and I can handle anything that comes my way.

Episode XIII

"Into every woman's life a little diamond should fall"

Regardless where you stand in life; you should try to shine like a diamond. What I mean by that is taking time to come out your comfort zone and network with a group of individuals you have never engaged with before and see what opportunities are offered. Your little diamond is that very gift/talent you have that can bring forth you are serving a larger population of diverse individuals that you were unaware could benefit from what you have to offer.

I recall serving as a certified volunteer within the community for two years helping others apply for jobs, mock interviews, resume building, and educational consulting when I needed the same help. I allowed my little diamonds to fall into the lives of others that needed more support than I did at the time and when the individuals return to share their success story about their job offer made me feel like I really made a positive impact in someone life. I kept the growth mindset while volunteering in the community. I knew one day that it would return one hundred-fold. I did not know that being apart of that community, I would meet the very two individuals who stepped in at anytime when I had a downfall professionally and personally. I met my personal growth coach and additional health advisor/survivor that guided me emotionally and socially through the process with my mother having stage four head and neck cancer. When I tell you that I gave all glory to God for lending me his angels! I never knew that years after my assignment volunteering; they would be humble and supportive to help me. As a woman with a growth mindset; those encounters I endured through various pressure points in my life allowed a multitude of diamonds fall into my path of success.

Episode XIV

"Everybody wants to be a diamond, but very few are willing to get cut"

It is everyone intentions to grow with time accomplishing the basic ideal written goals such as furthering their education, landing the right job that will place you in a different tax bracket, meeting the right person to share your life with, and make life all worth all that you have invested in it. All the want's that most individuals desire according to something they saw modeled elsewhere is hard work. Think to yourself; are you willing to put in the real time and dedication? Better yet; can you handle beginning from the bottom of the barrel with your gifts, talents, and capabilities or you just want to jump right in it?

Individuals with a growth mindset understand that there is a process. Most importantly; success is a major investment. You must invest your time, money, and opportunity to perfect your craft by giving back through community service. The pressure of success comes with rejection. Rejection feels like a paper cut. It hurts whether it's touched directly or indirectly. It's an uncomfortable feeling that causes you to be alert of how you handle things moving forward.

I have been rejected and told no many times knowing I could execute the opportunities I was pursuing. I have been cut down with words from friends, family, professionals, and outsiders due to my approach of handling business is firm but fair. To my understanding; its business over pleasure. I like to get things done and get it done the right way especially when other people may be affected by the decisions that are being made. I have lost some supporters and I have gained some supporters. It took some time for me to realize that road to success is a lonely place but a great place for you as the expert to plan and execute your goals and aspirations accordingly. To experience the royalties of being a diamond; you must accept the firm pressure and deep wombs. A diamond is formed and polished by going through the process.

Episode XV

"A diamond is a chunk of coal that did well under pressure"

Understand that you are not your address. Blaming your upbringing as to why you speak the way you do, dress the way you dress, and approach life the way you do is not always acceptable depending on circumstances. Many successful individual's upbringing was like a mass of coal; hard and dark with many ridged edges and cuts but they conquered. They conquered because they were determined not to relive the past and create a successful future for their families. They underwent the pressure and force from all angles of opposition and found their way to the mountain top.

 Through the stages of defining myself as a young scholar in undergraduate school; my first test of feeling the pressure was conceiving a child out of wedlock, following getting married and divorcing, and back to being a single mother again within a two year time period. I was negatively looked upon because from the outside; it looked as if I abandoned my marriage and did not give it any chances. That's not the case. My mindset was a little different being the go-getter that I am. The pressure became tense when I chose to live in a disclosed location without my children for two months because I did not have anything. It felt like I was doing visitations with my kids between my mother and grandmothers house. Soon as I got a job opportunity after losing my certified home child care facility by the state of North Carolina in result of separating from my at the time husband; I was able to become financially secured to locate an operating vehicle, a place for my children and I to stay, and began coming out the valley of fear, disappointment, bitterness, and shame. I didn't attend church for about two months so to return out the blue with the saints greeting you with hugs and questions that you really did not feel like answering because the damage was already done was too much pressure but I stood the test and conquered once again with a smile on my face. With all the pressure points compiled together; it taught me enough about trust and seeing others for whom they are. Most importantly; it taught me that I can remain successful despite any personal or professional limitations that come my way.

Episode XVI

"Some people lose diamonds in search of stones"

During the course of becoming the person one desire to be; having others to accept the talents and gifts that are offered on multiple platforms is expected when matriculating from one milestone to another. It is often seen that society chose to maneuver and decide on their next move in a way that it benefit all significant stakeholders that are involved. In some cases the decision can be the right decision for the moment or it could be the right decision for a lifetime; only time will tell. A person interest in contributing to another person and their goals or an organization can be sincere and impactful but that individual was chosen. When any diamond is traded for a stone; it will not retrieve the same amount of value the diamond added to the platform.

    I have not always been chosen and that's ok. I have applied for the six figure jobs in other states and have been offered multiple positions; however, due to being a single parent of two boys, just picking up and leaving is not so easy. I have applied for the same six figure jobs in my current city and surrounding areas and have not been offered one position. I recall teaching at a higher institution of learning during the beginning of my journey as a college professor and yearning to be effective in and outside the classroom. All of my observations were proficient and tasks that I was implementing within the classroom were being brought to the department chair to implement throughout the entire department as a mandatory end of the year project for all first time students. I had the dean to observe and select the best student creative t-shirt that advertised the institutions quality education plans that was selected to be the gear to drive the institution to success and decrease retention rates. With the sponsorship relationships that I create with all my adult learners as well as the dedication and passion I put into my work in adult education; when I pursued a leadership position, another individual was selected. I knew I qualified and was knowledgeable about the position and executed my interview with the best practices to fulfill all required duties and responsibilities. Later, I discovered that I was the only African American woman who applied; I was running up against my boss, and I was the only person who was pursuing a doctoral degree. In the political world; I was considered a curtesy interviewee. The institution had to fulfill their demographical requirements within the system so it would not be viewed as a bias selection process. Of course the institution later discovered that they traded a diamond for a stone and their goal for driving the student success rate did not increase in the capacity that was projected. People and opportunities will continue to loose diamonds searching for stones just to get by or find the cheapest and easy way out. Be that diamond!

Episode XVII

"Start living your life fearlessly; like a diamond"

It take more than one life experience to learn how to humble oneself and accept others and life the way it is. More than one life experience will also teach a person how to properly associate oneself with others without falling into the trap of false friendship advertisements and professional opportunities that sale you a dream of growth and wealth. Living life fearlessly like a diamond is accepting where you are in life and do what you can for the moment stress free. Maintaining a peace of mind throughout your daily routine is a great time to begin living your life fearlessly; like a diamond!

After sitting on my psychologist couch with a box of tissue retelling my childhood up until my adulthood as a parent, educator, coach, and mentor brought clarity to why my body was tired and shut down. It took ten days to accept society's personal bill of rights and apply to every person, association, organization, and community member that I came in contact with; past or present. If I did not want to answer my cell phone; I did not answer. If I did not want to go to an event; I did not go. I learned to not feel like I had to explain myself when I made a decision that was best for me. At this point; I was living my life fearlessly; like a diamond! I was fearless of the status of the relationship I had at the time, friendships that I thought were trustworthy, and decisions that would benefit my mental health. I begin cleaning my plate so that I could properly manage my life and priorities. When the wise men often say that *"the mind is a terrible thing to waste"*; truth is an understatement. I did not lose my mind; my mind was drained from the persistence and endurance while traveling the road of success. My doctor advised me to train my body to rest at times to gain energy and allow my mental to gain strength. Practice make perfect as society believes. I practice resting, saying no to large commitments, being on every set, and chasing friendships/relationships in order to feel complete. I no longer have the fear of being alone. I embrace my alone time with our without a significant other or friend. I'm convinced that

I have practice being alone so much; it's becoming challenging to get out and be the extrovert I truly am. When you are transitioning into God's own image; you have no choice but to comply, be humble, learn, and listen. Remember; living life fearlessly; like a diamond begin with *you*.

Episode XVIII

"You can't rush something you want to last forever"

Think about that very thing that you desire; whether it's success within your career or on your job, the perfect spouse, and/or the newest Mercedes Benz because you know you deserve it and you must have it right now. Do note that everything you desire comes with a step by step procedure or protocol. Most importantly; are you in the right position to gain those things that you yearn for? Do you know what it takes to maintain what you desire? Do you honestly think it's safe to rush something you want to last forever?

We have all been in the position where we are forcing things during the wrong season in our lives; then we are upset because things did not go as planned. As I grew older and much wiser; I understand the importance of waiting for what I desire so that once it's retrieved; I will be in the right position to maintain the yearnings of my heart. Most importantly; the desires of your heart will appear when your least expected to accept them. Do not feed into the social clock that society has created and its expectations for what supposed to happen in your life at a certain time period.

My social clock was all backwards. I conceived two children out of wedlock, been divorced, and happily dating while effectively co-parenting with my children's father. Through all the barriers; I never gave up on my goals and aspirations to be an effective and passionate educator, mentor, and coach for the next generation. There are somethings on my wish list that I want to happen before my late thirties and nope it's not a baby!..lol In due time; all things will come to past.

Episode XIX

"Better a diamond with a flaw than a pebble without"

Even successful people have flaws. They are not perfect human beings. They get tired, aggravated, upset, and want to throw in the towel from time to time; however, they embrace the importance for pursuing their purpose. Being a diamond is not mainly what you look like when you walk out the door in the mornings. Being a diamond is demonstrated by enduring the fire and pressure in order to accomplish whatever that's place in front of you. Looking poised and on point with dramatic eye lashes, a duffle bag, pearls, and red bottoms comes after the rigorous journey. Pop out when the job is done! Pepples don't shine like a diamond. Even in your toughest times; you should still illuminate the room with your gifts and talents.

This diamond here; yes I called myself a diamond because I have been there, done that, been broken down, and back pursuing my passion does not mind sharing one major flaw that I have and currently working to overcome as I continue to surround myself with great people. I am whole heartily an extrovert; meaning, I love interacting with people in general. It's not hard for me to strike up a conversation with someone where we share the same interest or viewpoint on something. However; going out my way in this present day to hold a friendship in any form or association is so hard to do due to past hurts and failures. My flaw is assuming that every person that's trying to get to know me has a hidden agenda and I do not feel comfortable or have the energy to find out therefore; I shut down. When invited to things that require me to fully engage is a challenge but it does completely stop me from pursuing my purpose. He's still smoothing out the edges and polishing my purpose!

Episode XX

"I love diamond facials; they leave me glowing and refreshed"

Your approach and image is another person first impression of who you really are. When you enter a room of unknown faces; what do you desire for them to perceive? Attitude, anger, bitterness, bourgeoisie or poised, passionate, persistent? Yes; a diamond shine bright but it does not blind the gifts, talents, and abilities of others.

My first official diamond facial was professionally performed by *makeupby_lesliemarie*. The diamond facial was to represent the process of the value of coal that was endured when mastering my final educational milestone August 2015. The total experience during my professional diamond facial was filled with women empowerment. The professional artist and I shared valuable resources that would help each other excel in our own gifts, talents, and abilities. Many of our encounters have brought us to where we currently stand manifesting within our purpose. My goal during all of our encounters were to encourage and promote her profession as a certified make-up artist because every appointment provided a diamond experience that left me glowing and refreshed!

I recall sharing one of my professional portraits in my doctoral regalia and immediate reactions were directed towards the diamond facial that left me glowing and refreshed. Two years later; I still gain recognition for the marvelous work *makeupby_lesliemarie* performed for a special day of honor. I honor the gift she has bestowed within to make many memorable moments for various special occasions I had to prepare for. Most importantly; I honor the iron sharpening iron collaborations that we have experienced over the years. I do indeed look forward to establishing new memories and having diamond facials with *makeupby_lesliemarie* that leaves me glowing and refreshed to pursue my purpose and passion.

Episode XXI

"Be careful who you cast your diamonds too"

Be alert who you share your vision with. Everyone that's cheering for you can be plotting behind you. Remember when your vision was crafted together and you had it on paper and you needed to share it with one person just to get confirmation that you were moving in the right direction? That very person you know that's going to be there to support you immediately begin asking question after question seeking information on how you crafted your thoughts to implement your vision. While you're pouring out all your pearls to your ride or die and others may say ace boom coon; they are finding a way to include themselves in your purpose with little to no effort with the hard labor that's required. It's imperative that your pearls (vision, mission, purpose) be held close and only shared with those who have the resources to cast your pearls that produce positive results. Casting your pearls via social media and with everyone you come in contact with is considered a dream killer. Your pearls are not for everyone; therefore, be careful who you cast your pearls too.

    I recall assuming that everyone that called me friend, sister, Soror, or boo thang had my best interests in heart. The one person I thought would be there to support my goals and aspirations provided me with the shock of my life when it was time to show support by only being present. Another time was when I called one of my professional colleagues to share a vision and after I got the first couple of sentences out; the individual begin giving their input and how they would do it if they were to put your project together. The next conversation began with *"I was thinking about doing something similar but with a twist"*. It's nothing wrong supporting a friend or professional colleague; however, you may have given them every tool needed to bring their vision, mission, and passion to life when you retrieved your resources through research, observation, and coaching from another scholar that's proficient in the area you are pursuing to manifest your purpose.

Episode XXII

"We are diamonds were gonna shine forever"

Depending on how much you value yourself and the production of your success will determine how long you are willing to be located in the coal mine. The coal mine is the outlier where the access includes experiencing underground operations with drifts, inclines, or spillways. Within the coal mine you will have to ask yourself if you can take the heat and pressure. It gets hot, overwhelming, and breathtaking. Blood, sweat, tears will transpire as you are carrying loads of coal through the drifts, inclines, and spillways to transform into diamond crystals. Your pieces of coal endure extensive heat and pressure; therefore your diamond (s) should have the four C's: color, clarity, cut, and carat weight. Quality is the international language for examining the superiority of any diamond. We as women desire to shine forever!

Accepting my medical diagnosis and dealing with daily challenges to overcome anxiety and depression when things trigger the psyche can be embarrassing and overwhelming. It take so much energy to tackle things that you were once familiar with not knowing if it or the environment could offset your feelings, actions, and approach to handling certain tasks the appropriate way; however, *"It Can Be Done"!* I was determined to get back on my feet and pursue the platform where I once stood motivating and inspiring others to achieve their goals and aspirations. Despite the coal mine experience; I had a strong and understanding support system that prayed, pushed, and proclaimed strength into my life to get me to this place. They often reminded me who I was when I felt unaccomplished and unworthy due to life's realities. I humbly accept the things I have endured because they taught me valuable and unforgettable lessons that will constantly remind me of the importance of mental health and the epidemic it has on society and the African American culture. I stand to share that it is ok to seek professional help and be a prominent scholar in your local community. It's more embarrassing to not seek help to deal with daily challenges while help, aiding, and assisting others and face a major pitfall that takes even more time to overcome due to the process of overcoming mental health illnesses.

How would you best reveal your diamond that's within? Are you and your capabilities cut like a marquise, princess, pear, oval, heart, or emerald? An unknown philosopher once stated; *"everyone is gifted, but most people never open their package"*. Open the box; and *shine forever like a diamond!* As always; *"continue to be a beacon of light"*.

www.ingramcontent.com/pod-product-compliance
Lightning Source LLC
Chambersburg PA
CBHW031549210526
45464CB00003B/1217